Superfood Cookbook
Delicious Healthy Superfoods Food Recipes Clean Eating

Table of Contents

Introduction	5
Chapter 1: Breakfast Recipes	8
PowerHouse Smoothie	8
Sweet Potato Hash	8
Sweet Potato Toast	9
Berry and Kefir Smoothie	10
Blueberry Overnight Oatmeal	10
Sweet Potato-Encrusted Quiches	11
Chia-Blueberry Pudding	12
Cherry-Oatmeal Smoothie	12
Chocolate and Banana Sweet Potato Toast	13
Chocolate Chia Pudding	13
Chia and Quinoa Oatmeal	14
Peanut Butter and Apple Smoothie	15
Mango and Coconut Chia Pudding	15
Berry Cauliflower Smoothie	16
Apple, Cinnamon, and Quinoa Bowl	16
Flower-Power Oatmeal	17
Cold Cereal with Berries	17
Watermelon Salad	18
Chapter 2: Lunch Recipes	19
Tuna and Avocado on Sweet Potato Toast	19
Spaghetti Squash with Tomatoes and Almond Pesto	19
Chickpea Quinoa Bowl	21
Farro, Kale, and Squash Salad	22

Lentil and Vegetable Salad	24
White Bean and Tuna Wrap	25
Chicken and Minestrone Soup	26
Fish Casserole	27
Pinto Bean Burgers	28
Veggie Primavera	29
Bean and Turkey Chili	30
Fruit and Chicken Curry	31
Vegetable Stir-Fry	32
Vegetable Gyro	33
Avocado and Goat Cheese on Toast	34
Barley and Avocado Bowl	34
Baked Eggs in Avocados	35
Avocado Fingers	36
Chapter 3: Dinner Recipes	37
Broccoli and Salmon	37
Broccoli, Feta, and Quinoa Salad	38
Salmon Salad	39
Chicken and Broccoli Salad	40
Sea Bass and Beetroot Salsa	41
Salmon and Crème Fraiche Pasta	42
Turkey and Lemon Meatballs	43
Sesame-encrusted Salmon	44
Roasted vegetables with honey and feta cheese	45
Tomato and Mango Curry	46
Creamy Salmon Tagliatelle	47
Salmon Stir-Fry	48

Salmon Bake	49
Egg-fried rice with Mushroom and salmon	50
Coriander and Chickpea Salad	51
Beat and Bean Salad	52
Roasted Cauliflower and Oranges	53
Roasted lemon and parsnips	54
Conclusion	55

© Copyright 2018 by Charlie Mason - All rights reserved.

The following Book is reproduced below with the goal of providing information that is as accurate and reliable as possible. Regardless, purchasing this Book can be seen as consent to the fact that both the publisher and the author of this book are in no way experts on the topics discussed within and that any recommendations or suggestions that are made herein are for entertainment purposes only. Professionals should be consulted as needed prior to undertaking any of the action endorsed herein.

This declaration is deemed fair and valid by both the American Bar Association and the Committee of Publishers Association and is legally binding throughout the United States.

Furthermore, the transmission, duplication or reproduction of any of the following work including specific information will be considered an illegal act irrespective of if it is done electronically or in print. This extends to creating a secondary or tertiary copy of the work or a recorded copy and is only allowed with an expressed written consent from the Publisher. All additional rights reserved.

The information in the following pages is broadly considered to be a truthful and accurate account of facts, and as such any inattention, use or misuse of the information in question by the reader will render any resulting actions solely under their purview. There are no scenarios in which the publisher or the original author of this work can be in any fashion deemed liable for any hardship or damages that may befall them after undertaking the information described herein.

Additionally, the information in the following pages is intended only for informational purposes and should thus be thought of as universal. As befitting its nature, it is presented without assurance regarding its prolonged validity or interim quality. Trademarks that are mentioned are done without written consent and can in no way be considered an endorsement from the trademark holder.

Introduction

Congratulations on purchasing The *Superfood Cookbook* and thank you for doing so.

The following chapters will discuss all recipes you can prepare in less than one hour. This book is intended to help educate you on the benefits of incorporating more superfoods. When you eat food, it is the best thing you can do for your body to ingest the most nutritious fuel possible.

There are plenty of books on this subject on the market, thanks again for choosing this one! Every effort was made to ensure it is full of as much useful information as possible, please enjoy!

Superfoods are defined as nutrient-dense foods with copious amounts of vitamins and minerals. These foods help us to be healthy and live longer, richer and fuller lives. People from all stages of life can benefit from the consumption of these super-healthy foods. Whether you are pregnant, a child, older than 50, or are just needing an extra energy boost, everyone needs extra vitamins.

If you are pregnant, some superfoods that are extremely beneficial are:
- Eggs
- Berries
- Yogurt
- Whole grains
- Sweet potatoes
- Legumes
- Broccoli
- Seafood

If you are over 50, superfoods that can be beneficial are:
- Salmon
- Oranges
- Broccoli
- Dark leafy greens

If you have children, the best superfoods for them to consume are:
- Berries
- Seafood
- Seeds
- Leafy greens
- Nut butters and Nuts
- Orange vegetables and fruit
- Whole grains
- Yogurt
- Oatmeal

Perhaps you are a perfectly healthy adult who just needs extra energy for the daily grind. Here are some foods for you to try, besides coffee:

- Oatmeal
- Quinoa
- Blueberries
- Salmon
- Avocados
- Goji Berries
- Almonds
- Lentils
- Kale

Every recipe in this book is healthful and delicious. No matter what kind of shape your health is in, these recipes are for you.

As a way of saying thank you for purchasing my book, please use your link below to claim your 3 FREE Cookbooks on Health, Fitness & Dieting Instantly

https://bit.ly/2Lvj2Pm

You can also share your link with your friends and families whom you think that can benefit from the cookbooks or you can forward them the link as a gift!

Chapter 1: Breakfast Recipes

PowerHouse Smoothie

Ingredients:

- Chia Seeds (1 Tablespoon)
- Almond Butter (1 Tablespoon)
- Coconut oil (1 Tablespoon)
- Plant-Based Milk (1 cup)
- Kale (1.5 cups, packed)
- Banana (.5 of one)

Preparation:

- Blend all the ingredients until smooth in a high-speed blender.

Sweet Potato Hash

Ingredients:

- Salt and Pepper
- Parsley (For Decoration)
- Cumin (.5 teaspoon)
- Olive Oil (2 Tablespoons)
- Eggs (4 Large)
- Bell Peppers (.5 each red and yellow, chopped)
- Onion (1 medium, chopped)
- Sweet Potatoes (2 cups, uncooked)

Preparation:

- Set the oven to broil.
- Use an oven safe skillet to warm the olive oil. Once hot, add in the onions and sweet potatoes.

- Cook for approximately seven minutes. Add bell peppers and spices.
- Cook for an additional five to seven minutes, occasionally stirring.
- Proceed to crack the eggs atop the hash mixture, and then place the skillet in the oven on the middle rack underneath the broiler.
- Cook until eggs are to preference.
- Serve with parsley.

Sweet Potato Toast

Ingredients:

- Frank's Hot Sauce (.5 teaspoon)
- Chives (.5 teaspoon)
- Egg (1 large, poached or fried)
- Spinach (.33 cups spinach, cooked)
- Sweet potato (1 Large, sliced .25 inches thick)

Preparation:

- Toast a slice of sweet potato in a toaster or in the oven until barely turning brown, approximately 13 minutes.
- Top with egg, spinach, chives, and hot sauce.

Berry and Kefir Smoothie

Ingredients:

- Vanilla Extract (.5 teaspoon)
- Almond Butter (2 teaspoons)
- Banana (.5 of one, ripe)
- berries (1.5 cups, mixed or single kind, frozen)
- Kefir (1 cup, plain)

Preparation:

- Combine every ingredient into a blender.
- Blend until smooth.

Blueberry Overnight Oatmeal

Ingredients:

- Maple Syrup (2 teaspoons)
- Pecans (1 Tablespoon, chopped)
- Yogurt (2 Tablespoons)
- Blueberries (.5 cups, frozen or fresh)
- Salt (Pinch)
- Water (.5 Cups)
- Oatmeal (.5 cups, old-fashioned rolled)

Preparation:

- Throw oats, water, and salt into jar.
- Cover and refrigerate overnight.
- In the morning, top with the remaining ingredients.

Sweet Potato-Encrusted Quiches

Ingredients:

- Milk (.5 cups, plant-based)
- Eggs (6, large)
- Cheese (1 cup, shredded
- Bell Pepper (.5, red, chopped)
- Avocado Oil (1 Tablespoon)
- Sweet Potato (1.5 cups, peeled and shredded)

Preparation:

- Preheat oven to 350 degrees Fahrenheit. Use a cooking spray or Canola Oil to coat a muffin tin.
- Throw sweet potato and toss in oil in a bowl. Divide the mixture equally amongst the muffin tins. Press down the bottoms and side to form the crust.
- Divide the bell pepper chunks and then sprinkle with cheese.
- In a measuring cup or bowl, whisk together the milk, eggs, salt, and pepper. Proceed to divide mixture into all the muffin cups.
- Bake for approximately 25 minutes.
- Remove the quiches with a knife and scrape all around the sides while they are still fresh out of the oven.

Chia-Blueberry Pudding

Ingredients:

- Almonds (1 Tablespoon, slivers)
- Blueberries (.5 cup, frozen or fresh)
- Almond Extract (.125 teaspoon)
- Maple Syrup (2 teaspoons)
- Chia seeds (2 Tablespoons)
- Milk (.5 cup, plant-based)

Preparation:

- Combine milk, chia seeds, syrup, and almond extract in a bow.
- Cover and chill for eight hours, or up to three days.
- When ready to eat, add blueberries and almonds.

Cherry-Oatmeal Smoothie

Ingredients:

- Ice-cubes (.5 cup, small)
- Honey (1 Tablespoon)
- Black Cherries (.5 cup, frozen or fresh)
- Strawberries (.75 cup, fresh or frozen)
- Milk (.5 cup, plant-based)
- Oatmeal (.33 cup, Quick, rolled)

Preparation:

- In a microwave-safe bowl, combine the oatmeal and water and stir in half of the milk.
- Microwave for 40 seconds, or until oatmeal is tender. Cool for a couple of minutes.

- In a blender, combine the microwaved oatmeal along with the rest of the ingredients, stopping at honey.
- Blend until smooth. Add the ice, blend until smooth again.

Chocolate and Banana Sweet Potato Toast

Ingredients:

- Cereal (1 teaspoon, crispy)
- Banana (1, sliced in half, lengthwise)
- Chocolate-Hazelnut Spread (1 Tbsp)
- Sweet Potato (1, cut in .25-inch slices)

Preparation:

- Toast the sweet potato in a toaster or oven until barely cooked through and brown. This will take about 13 minutes.
- Once out of the oven, top with the spread, banana, and cereal.

Chocolate Chia Pudding

Ingredients:

- Almonds (1 Tablespoon, sliced)
- Chia Seeds (2 Tablespoons)
- Raspberries (.5 cup, fresh or frozen)
- Vanilla Extract (.25 teaspoon)
- Cacao (.5 teaspoon, Raw)
- Maple Syrup (2 Tablespoons)
- Milk (.5 cup, plant-based)

Preparation:

- Combine, milk, chia seeds, cacao, maple syrup, and vanilla together in a bowl.
- Cover and chill in the refrigerator for at least eight hours up to three days.
- When ready to eat, top the pudding with raspberries and almonds.

Chia and Quinoa Oatmeal

Ingredients:

- Salt (.75 teaspoon)
- Cinnamon (1 teaspoon)
- Chia or Hemp seeds (.5 cup)
- Fruit (1 cup, raisins or cranberries, dried)
- Quinoa (1 cup, any variety)
- Oatmeal (2 cups, Old-Fashioned, Rolled)

Preparation:

- To make the dry mix: Throw all the ingredients into an airtight container.
- To prepare one serving of the hot cereal: Add 1.25 cups of milk or water to 0.33 cup of oatmeal mixture in a saucepan. Bring the mixture to a boil.
- Partially covered, reduce the heat to low and simmer. Stir the mixture occasionally until it thickened for about 12 minutes.
- Turn off the stove and let the mixture rest for five minutes while covered.

Peanut Butter and Apple Smoothie

Ingredients:

- Ice Cubes (5)
- Cinnamon (.25 teaspoon, ground)
- Vanilla Extract (1 Teaspoon)
- Honey (2 teaspoons)
- Peanut butter (2 Tablespoons)
- Apple (1, small, chopped)
- Milk (1 cup, plant-based)

Preparation:

- Throw all ingredients into a blender.
- Blend until smooth.

Mango and Coconut Chia Pudding

Ingredients:

- Coconut (1 Tablespoon, shredded)
- Mango (.5 cup, diced, fresh or frozen)
- Coconut Extract (.5 teaspoon)
- Maple Syrup (2 teaspoons)
- Chia Seeds (2 Tablespoons)
- Milk (.5 cup, plant-based)

Preparation:

- Combine milk, chia seeds, maple syrup, and extract of coconut in a bowl.
- Cover the bowl and chill for about eight hours to three days.
- When ready to eat, top with mango and coconut.

Berry Cauliflower Smoothie

Ingredients:

- Milk (2 cups, unsweetened plant-based)
- Maple syrup (2 teaspoons)
- Banana (1 cup, chopped)
- Berries (.5 cup, mixed, frozen)
- Cauliflower (1 cup, riced)

Preparation

- Throw all ingredients into a blender.
- Blend until smooth, about three minutes.

Apple, Cinnamon, and Quinoa Bowl

Ingredients:

- Honey (.5 teaspoon)
- Almonds (4 teaspoons sliced)
- Salt (.125 teaspoons)
- Cinnamon (.25 teaspoon, ground)
- Quinoa (.25 cup, any variety)
- Apple (.66 cup, diced)
- Milk (.75 cup, plant-based)

Preparation:

- Combine milk, 0.33 cup of apple, quinoa, cinnamon, and salt into a saucepan.
- Bring to boil then simmer. Cover until the liquid is absorbed approximately 11-12 minutes.
- Remove from heat and let it rest for about five minutes.
- Top with the remaining ingredients.

Flower-Power Oatmeal

Ingredients:

- Raspberry (1)
- Blueberries (15)
- Mango (5, slices)
- Maple Syrup (1 teaspoon)
- Oatmeal (.5 cup, old-fashioned, rolled)
- Milk (1 cup, non-dairy)

Preparation:

- Throw oatmeal into a saucepan along with milk. Boil the oatmeal over medium-high heat.
- Simmer and stir often for approximately five minutes until thickened.
- Add maple syrup.
- Put oatmeal in a bowl, and then use the rest of the ingredients to make a flower.

Cold Cereal with Berries

Ingredients:

- Milk (.75 cup, plant-based)
- Goji Berries (.125 cup)
- Strawberries (.125 cup, frozen or fresh)
- Cheerios (1 cup)

Preparation:

- Combine all ingredients into a bowl.
- Enjoy!

Watermelon Salad

Ingredients:

- Chia Seeds (1 Tablespoon)
- Coconut (.25 cup, shredded)
- Blueberries (.5 cup, frozen or fresh)
- Watermelon (1 cup, diced)
- Lime Juice (Splash)

Preparation:

- Throw together all the ingredients in a bowl.
- Top with a splash of lime juice.

Chapter 2: Lunch Recipes

Tuna and Avocado on Sweet Potato Toast

Ingredients:

- Sesame seeds (.125 teaspoon, toasted)
- Nori (.5 teaspoon, slivered)
- Tuna (1 Tablespoon, flaked)
- Ginger (1 Tablespoon, pickled, chopped)
- Carrot (1 Tablespoon, julienned)
- Avocado (.25 of one, mashed)
- Sweet Potato (1 slice, .25 inch thick)

Preparation:

- Toast sweet potato slice for at least 12 minutes or until lightly browned and thoroughly cooked.
- Top with remaining ingredients.

Spaghetti Squash with Tomatoes and Almond Pesto

Ingredients:

Almond Pesto

- Water (.25 cup)
- Olive Oil (.25 cup, Extra Virgin)
- Salt (pinch)
- Pepper (pinch)
- Vinegar (1.5 Tablespoon, Red Wine)
- Garlic (1 clove)
- Almonds (.33 cup, raw)
- Parmesan Cheese (.5 cup, grated)
- Parsley (1 cup, fresh)
- Basil (2 cups, fresh)

Spaghetti Squash with Other Vegetables

- Cannellini Beans (1 cup, rinsed and drained)
- Pepper (pinch)
- Salt (pinch)
- Grape Tomatoes (2 pints, halved)
- Water (.25 cup)
- Spaghetti Squash (1, 3-pound)

Preparation:

To make the Pesto:

- Pulse basil, parsley, parmesan, garlic, almonds, pepper, and salt into a food processor until coarsely chopped.
- Add in olive oil and then blend until combined well.
- Add water, pulse to mix well.

To prepare vegetables:

- Preheat oven to 400 degrees Fahrenheit.
- Place an aluminum foil into a baking sheet.
- Cut in half and lengthwise the squash before scooping out seeds. Place open side down in a microwave-safe dish with water.
- Heat the microwave for about 15 minutes or until flesh can be scraped off with a fork.

- Toss the tomatoes in oil, pepper, and salt in a bowl. Move them to the baking sheet and roast for 10-11 minutes until wrinkled and soft.
- Remove from the oven, add in beans, and stir.
- Scrape spaghetti squash flesh into a bowl and top with tomato and bean mixture, along with pesto.

Chickpea Quinoa Bowl

Ingredients:

- Parsley (2 Tablespoons, chopped)
- Feta Cheese (.25 cup, crumbled)
- Cucumber (1 cup, diced)
- Chickpeas (1 15-ounce can, rinsed and drained)
- Onion (.25 cup, red, finely chopped)
- Olives (.25 cup, Kalamata, chopped)
- Quinoa (2 cups, cooked)
- Cumin (.5 teaspoon)
- Paprika (1 teaspoon)
- Garlic (1 clove)
- Olive Oil (4 Tablespoons, Extra Virgin)
- Almonds (.25 cup, slivered)
- Bell Peppers (1 jar, small, rinsed)

Preparation:

- Throw peppers, almonds, half of olive oil, garlic, and cumin into a food processor. Process until smooth.
- Mix quinoa, olives, onion, and the other half of olive oil into a bowl
- To serve, divide into bowls, top with chickpeas, feta, and parsley.

Farro, Kale, and Squash Salad

Ingredients:

Farro
- Salt (pinch)
- Water (1.5 cups)
- Farro (.75 cup)

Squash
- Pepper(pinch)
- Salt(pinch)
- Olive Oil (1 Tablespoon, Extra Virgin)
- Butternut Squash (4 cups, .5-inch cubes)

Kale
- Garlic (3 cloves, minced)
- Vinegar (5 Tablespoons, red wine)
- Olive oil (7 Tablespoons, Extra Virgin)
- Pepitas (.25 cup, toasted)
- Feta cheese (.5 cup, crumbled)
- Salt (pinch
- Pepper(pinch)
- Mustard (1 Tablespoon, Dijon)
- Water (1.25 cups)
- Kale (8 ounces)

Preparation:

- Preheat oven to 425 degrees Fahrenheit. Use cooking oil to coat a baking sheet.
- To make the Farro: toast the Farro until fragrant or for approximately two minutes over medium heat in a saucepan.
- Add salt and water. Boil.
- For 30 minutes, cover and simmer the Farro. Drain, then fluff with a fork.
- To make the Squash: Throw Squash together with salt, pepper, and oil.
- Spread out the squash on a baking sheet and roast for about 25 minutes.
- To make the Kale: Toss six tablespoons of olive oil, mustard, vinegar, pepper, and salt. Cut stems off kale then slice leaves into strips.
- Add to bowl and mix the dressing well with kale.
- On medium heat, heat the last of the oil in a skillet. Add stems from kale as well as salt and pepper.
- Occasionally stir for one to two minutes until slightly charred.
- Add .25 cup of water, cover, then cook for two minutes.
- Repeat four or five times.
- Transfer stems to cutting board, slice into pieces.
- Assemble all the ingredients together.

Lentil and Vegetable Salad

Ingredients:

- Kale (2 cups, thinly sliced)
- Lettuce (8 cups)
- Garlic (1 clove, Quartered)
- White miso (1.5 teaspoons)
- Lemon Juice (1 Tablespoon)
- Buttermilk (.25 cup)
- Mayonnaise (.33 cup)
- Tarragon (.5 cup, fresh, chopped)
- Chives (.5 cup, fresh, chopped)
- Parsley (.5 cup, fresh, chopped)
- Lentils (.75 cup, green)
- Pepper (pinch)
- Salt(pinch)
- Olive Oil (1 Tablespoon, Extra Virgin)

- Green Beans (2 cups)
- Broccoli (4 cups, florets)

Preparation:

- Preheat oven to 400 degrees Fahrenheit
- Combine green beans, broccoli, oil, salt, and pepper on a cookie sheet.
- Roast for about 20 minutes, stirring once.
- Boil lentils and water over high heat. Simmer, cover, and then cook for about 25 minutes until tender.
- Rinse and drain.
- Blend herbs, mayonnaise, buttermilk, lemon juice, miso, salt, garlic, and pepper in a food processor or blender until smooth.
- Toss lettuce with dressing, vegetable, and lentils.

White Bean and Tuna Wrap

Ingredients:

- Carrots (sticks)
- Cucumber (sticks)
- Tortilla Wraps (6)
- Parsley (.25 cup, minced)
- Tomatoes (1 cup, cherry, sliced)
- Tuna (2 6-ounce cans, plain, flaked)
- Cannellini Beans (2 15-ounce cans, rinsed, drained, mashed)
- Olive Oil (2 Tablespoons, Extra Virgin)
- Pepper (pinch)
- Salt (pinch)
- Onion (3 Tablespoon, minced)
- Lemon Juice (2 Tablespoons)

Preparation:

- Whisk together onion, olive oil, lemon juice, salt, and pepper in a small bowl.
- Throw beans, tomatoes, tuna, and parsley in a bowl. Mix in the dressing.
- Put 0.75 cups of bean mixture in each tortilla.

Chicken and Minestrone Soup

Ingredients:

- Pasta (1 cup, cooked, small variety)
- Chicken (1 pound, cut into bite-size portions)
- Tomatoes (1 can, diced)
- Cannellini Beans (1 15-ounce can, rinsed and drained)
- Vegetables (1 pound, Italian, frozen)
- Chicken Broth (1 container)
- Italian Seasoning (.25 teaspoon)
- Garlic (2 cloves, minced)
- Olive Oil (2 Tablespoons, Extra Virgin)

Preparation:
- Over medium heat, heat up the oil in a large saucepan. Toss in garlic and Italian seasoning.
- Cook for 30 seconds, and then add in the broth, vegetables, beans, and tomatoes.
- Boil on high and reduce heat to simmer for seven minutes.
- Combine with chicken and cook for five minutes.
- Serve with pasta.

Fish Casserole

Ingredients:

- Parsley (.25 cup, chopped)
- Lemon Juice (2 Tablespoons)
- Tomatoes (2, deseeded, cut into .25-inch slices)
- Fish Filets (4, halibut or cod)
- Garlic (3 cloves, chopped)
- Salt (pinch)
- Pepper (pinch)
- Italian Peppers (2, large, sliced thin)
- Potatoes (1 pound, quartered)

- Olive Oil (2 Tablespoons)
- Olives (.25 cup, Kalamata)

Preparation:

- Preheat oven to 400 degrees Fahrenheit. Use one tablespoon of oil to coat a casserole dish.
- Lay the potatoes and pepper in the dish and add salt and pepper. Bake for 35 minutes.
- Toss garlic over the dish. Season fish filets with salt and pepper then lay on top of potatoes along with olives and tomatoes. Drizzle with olive oil and lemon juice. Top with parsley.
- Bake for 25 minutes.

Pinto Bean Burgers

Ingredients:

- Tomatoes (12 slices)
- Lettuce or Spinach
- Pita Bread (Halved)
- Tortilla Chips (.5 cup, crushed)
- Cumin (.5 teaspoon)
- Chili Powder (1 teaspoon)
- Egg (1 Large)

- Salsa (.5 cup)
- Bread Crumbs (.5 cup)
- Pinto Beans (2 15.5-ounce cans, rinsed and drained)

Preparation:

- Preheat broiler and coat cookie sheet with cooking spray.
- Put aside 1 cup of beans. Put remaining beans in a food processor.
- In a bowl, throw together the reserved beans, bread crumbs, egg, salsa, spices. Add the tortilla chips and processed beans.
- Mix together then form six patties. Spray both sides of patties with oil.
- Place about four inches from broiler, turning only once after 10 minutes. Serve in pita with remaining ingredients.

Veggie Primavera

Ingredients:

- Parsley (2 Tablespoons)
- Heavy Cream (3 Tablespoons)
- Salt (pinch)
- Pepper (pinch)
- Italian-Herb Seasoning (.25 teaspoon)

- Sugar (.5 teaspoon)
- Textured Vegetable Protein (.5 cup, follow directions on package)
- Tomato Sauce (1 small can)
- Tomatoes (1 can, stewed)
- Garlic (2 cloves, minced)
- Olive Oil (2 Tablespoons)
- Spaghetti Squash (1 4-pound)

Preparation:

- Cut squash in half, lengthwise. Put in a microwave-safe dish, open-side down in microwave for 20 minutes on high. Rotate once.
- Warm oil in a skillet over medium heat. Combine onion and garlic, and cook until softened for 10 minutes,
- Throw in the next seven ingredients. Reduce heat to simmer for 10 minutes.
- Add in cream, stir, and cook for two more minutes.
- Scrape squash onto a plate, top with sauce and parsley.

Bean and Turkey Chili

Ingredients:

- Rice (1.5 cups, cooked)
- Italian-style meatballs (1 pack, fully cooked)

- Kidney, Pinto, and Black Beans (1 Can of each, rinsed and drained)
- Oregano (.5 teaspoon)
- Cumin (.5 teaspoon)
- Salt (1 teaspoon)
- Chili Powder (1 Tablespoon)
- Tomato Sauce (1 can)
- Tomatoes (1 can, whole in juice)
- Garlic (3 cloves, minced)
- Sweet Pepper (1, green, chopped)
- Onion (1, chopped)
- Canola Oil (2 Tablespoon)

Preparation:

- Heat oil over medium heat in large saucepan. Toss in onion, garlic, and pepper.
- Cook and stir for about seven minutes.
- Throw in tomato sauce, chili powder, salt, cumin, and oregano. Break up all ingredients with wooden spoon. Continue to cook for five minutes.
- Add in beans and meatballs. Bring to a boil, reduce heat and cover for five minutes.
- Serve over rice.

Fruit and Chicken Curry

Ingredients:

- Salt (pinch)

- Canola oil (1 Tablespoon)
- Chicken Breasts (4, boneless and skinless)
- Cornstarch (1 teaspoon, mixed with 2 tablespoons cold water)
- Water (.5 cup)
- Orange juice (.25 cup)
- Pepper (.75 teaspoon)
- Cumin (.25 teaspoon)
- Curry powder (1 teaspoon)
- Banana (1)
- Pears (2, Red Bosc)
- Apples (2, granny Smith)

Preparation:

- Core apples and pears leaving the skin on and cut into cubes. Cut banana into 0.5-inch slices.
- Cook curry, cumin, and pepper in pan until fragrant. Add fruit juice and water.
- Boil, cover, and then reduce to simmer for 13 minutes,
- Add in cornstarch and cook for two more minutes.
- Preheat broiler, drizzle oil on chicken, and season with salt and pepper.
- Place chicken on cookie sheet four inches from broiler then cook for five minutes. Turn and continue to broil for three minutes.
- Transfer everything to a plate and can be served over rice.

Vegetable Stir-Fry

Ingredients:

- Cornstarch (1 Tablespoon)
- Onion (1, red, sliced thin)
- Bell pepper (1 medium red, sliced)
- Vegetables (12-ounces, frozen)
- Canola Oil (1 Tablespoon)
- Stir-fry Sauce (.5 cup, premade Kikkoman's)
- Chicken Breast (1 pound, boneless and skinless)

Preparation:

- Combine chicken and stir-fry sauce in a bowl.
- In a skillet, warm oil over medium heat. Add vegetables, onions, and pepper. Cook for eight minutes, and then remove from skillet. Take vegetables out and place aside.
- Throw the chicken in pan and cook for four minutes. Stir frequently, and then add the vegetables back to pan. Cook for another minute then serve.

Vegetable Gyro

Ingredients:

- Feta Cheese (1 package, garlic and herb)
- Tomatoes (2 large, sliced)
- Onion (.5 of one, sliced thin)
- Lettuce (.5 head, sliced)
- Pita Bread
- Salt (pinch)
- Pepper (pinch)
- Dill (1 Tablespoon)
- Lemon Juice (1 Tablespoon)
- Cucumber (.5 peeled, deseeded, diced)
- Yogurt (6-ounce package, low-fat, plain, drained)

Preparation:

Sauce
- Combine yogurt, garlic, lemon juice, cucumber, dill, salt, and pepper in a bowl. Cover and chill in the refrigerator for 30 minutes.

To assemble gyros:

- Wrap pita bread in damp paper towel and heat in the microwave for 20 seconds. Lay puffy sides down on plates.
- Evenly spread down the middle the lettuce, yogurt sauce, onion, tomatoes, and feta.
- Fold like a taco.

Avocado and Goat Cheese on Toast

Ingredients:

- Bread (4 slices)
- Avocado (1, ripened)
- Goat cheese (.25 cup, crumbled)
- Salt (pinch)
- Red pepper (1 teaspoon, flakes)
- Olive Oil

Preparation:

- Toast bread until crispy. Mash avocado and spread on all pieces of toast.
- Top with goat cheese and drizzle with olive oil and spices.

Barley and Avocado Bowl

Ingredients:

- Pepper (pinch)
- Avocado (1, ripened, peeled, chopped)
- Sea salt (pinch)
- Almonds (.25 cup, toasted, sliced)
- Queso (.33 cup)
- Bean sprouts (1 cup0
- Barley (.5 cup, cooked)

Lemon Yogurt Sauce
- Salt (pinch)
- Chives (1 Tablespoon)
- Lemon juice (1 teaspoon)
- Yogurt (.5 cup, plain, non-Greek)

Preparation:

- In a bowl, combine barley, cheese, sprouts, almonds, and salt. Mix them together.
- Whisk all ingredients in a different bowl to make the yogurt sauce together.
- Divide barley in two bowls. Top with avocado chunks and yogurt sauce.

Baked Eggs in Avocados

Ingredients:

- Chives (1 Tablespoon)
- Pepper (pinch)
- Eggs (4, large)
- Avocados (2, ripened)

Preparation:

- Preheat oven to 425 degrees Fahrenheit.
- Cut avocados in half and remove pits. Scoop 2 tablespoons out of each avocado so the egg can fit comfortably in each.
- Place avocados in a baking dish and crack each egg over each avocado half. Make sure the yolk goes in first, so the white can mold around the yolk.
- Bake for 15-20 minutes. Season with herbs and spices.

Avocado Fingers

Ingredients:

- Prosciutto (1 ounce)
- Chili powder (1 teaspoon)
- Salt (1 teaspoon)
- Pepper (1 teaspoon)
- Goat cheese (2 ounces)
- Lime juice (1 Tablespoon)
- Avocados (4, ripened, sliced, peeled)

Preparation:

- Toss avocado slices in a bowl with lime juice. Stuff the center of each avocado with goat cheese.
- Sprinkle with spices.
- Wrap each avocado slice with a thin slice of prosciutto until goat cheese is secure.

Chapter 3: Dinner Recipes

Broccoli and Salmon

Ingredients:

- Pepper (pinch)
- Salt (pinch)
- Dill (enough for garnish)
- Cream (.5 pint)
- Spring onions (4, thinly sliced)
- Butter (1 ounce)
- White wine (.25 pint)
- Salmon filet (8 ounce, skinless and boneless)
- Pasta (12 ounces, tagliatelle)
- Broccoli (10 ounces)

Preparation:

- Cook pasta for about 9 minutes or until in a pan of boiling salted water. Drain in a colander.
- While the pasta cooks, put salmon in a pan to fry. Add wine, pepper, and salt.
- Boil the salmon and simmer for five minutes until salmon is cooked.
- Move fish to a plate and flake it up with a fork. Increase the heat on the stove until the liquid is simmering and then reduced to three tablespoons.
- Wash the broccoli, trim the base of each stalk and then chop the florets into three-centimeter-long pieces.
- Add the butter to the wine, then the onions, and broccoli. Sauté for three minutes.
- Add cream and cover. Simmer for three minutes until broccoli is tender.
- Remove lid and stir in the salmon flakes. Season and taste. Add sauce to cooked pasta and then toss.

Broccoli, Feta, and Quinoa Salad

Ingredients:

- Top of Form
- quinoa (2 cups)
- broccoli (10 ounces)
- Mint (1 cup, chopped)
- feta cheese, (10 ounces, crumbled)
- pumpkin seeds (1 cup)
- pomegranate seeds (1 fruit's worth)
- Parsley (1 cup chopped)
- tomatoes (3 ripe, deseeded, chopped)
- spring onions (1 bunch, finely sliced)
- olive oil (3 Tablespoons, extra virgin)
- lemon juice (3 tablespoons)

Preparation:

- Prepare quinoa according to the package. Leave to cool in a bowl in the fridge.
- Meanwhile, the broccoli can be chopped into bite-size pieces and then boiled until tender for approximately five minutes. Set aside.
- Heat up a skillet and toast the pumpkin seed until crunchy. Remove from heat and set aside.
- Once the quinoa and broccoli have cooled down, combine with the feta cheese, pomegranate seeds, tomato, onions, herbs, lemon juice and oil.
- Season with salt and pepper. Toss everything together until well combined.

Salmon Salad

Ingredients:

- Orange (1 fruit)
- Seeds (1 Tablespoon, mixed variety: sunflower, pumpkin, etc.)
- Almonds (25 grams, chopped)
- Green Onion (2, sliced)
- Red chili (.5 of one, deseeded, chopped)
- Olive oil (1 Tablespoon)
- Salmon filets (200 grams, skinned)
- Broccoli (200 grams)

Preparation:

- Using a tiered steamer, boil water in the bottom. Place broccoli in the water and then lay the salmon on top of the steamer. Cook for three minutes until both broccoli and salmon is cooked.
- Remove both from heat, drain the broccoli and let the fish cool.
- Warm the oil in the skillet, sauté the chili, green onions, nuts, and mixed seeds for three minutes until golden brown.
- Using a grater, gather some zest from the half of the orange. Add to the skillet with some juice from a squeeze of the orange.
- Season with salt and pepper.
- Tear the salmon into flakes with a fork. Combine with broccoli and the nut and chili mixture.

Chicken and Broccoli Salad

Ingredients:

- Salt (pinch)
- Pepper (pinch)
- Pine nuts (1 ounce, toasted)
- Broccoli (7 ounces)
- Garlic (1 clove, crushed)
- Sunflower oil (1 Tablespoon)
- Greens (5 ounces, spinach or lettuce)
- Green onion (6, sliced)
- Tomatoes (5 ounces, cherry, halved)
- Lemon Zest (from one lemon)
- Tarragon (1 handful, chopped)
- Chicken breasts (4, skinless, boneless, cut into strips)

Preparation:

- Throw the chicken into a bowl. Add the tarragon, zest, salt, and pepper. Mix well. Marinate in fridge for a few hours.
- Prepare the dressing and set aside.
- In a bowl, place the greens, tomatoes, and onions. Season with pepper and salt.
- Warm the oil in a large skillet. Sauté the chicken for about nine minutes, turning often, until cooked through and golden.
- Combine the garlic at the last minute. Remove from heat, add the dressing and stir together. Make sure the chicken is well-coated, and any bits are scraped off the base of the pan.
- Boil the broccoli in water for five minutes until tender.

- Top the salad with chicken and broccoli. Garnish with pine nuts.

Sea Bass and Beetroot Salsa

Ingredients:

- Mint (2 Tablespoons, chopped)
- Lime Zest (2 limes)
- Green onions (6, sliced)
- Beetroot (8 ounces, cooked and chopped)
- Salt (to season)
- Pepper (to season)
- Bass Filets (4-6)
- Olive Oil (4 tablespoons)

Preparation:

- Heat the olive oil in skillet. Season the bass and proceed to sauté it, skin-side down, in two batches. Press the fillets down with a spatula and cook for approximately four minutes until the skin becomes crispy.
- Remove from heat but keep it warm.
- Wash the pan (remove the fish first) and add the rest of the oil, then the beetroot and heat it up over medium heat for approximately four minutes.
- Add the onion and lime zest. Stir in mint, then season to taste. Arrange two filets on a plate, then top with salsa.

Salmon and Crème Fraiche Pasta

Ingredients:

- Parsley (sprigs for Garnish)
- Pepper (pinch)
- Salt (pinch)
- Crème Fraiche (250 milliliters)
- Parsley (2 Tablespoons, chopped)
- Green Beans (6 ounces, trimmed, halved)
- Broccoli (4 ounces, small florets)
- Leek (1 large, trimmed, sliced)
- Pasta Shells (12 ounces)
- Salmon (418 grams, canned, wild pink)

Preparation:

- Drain the canned salmon, reserving three tablespoons of its liquid. Make sure there are no bones or any skin then break apart the salmon into chunks. Set aside.
- Cook the pasta according to the instructions and at the same time, cook the broccoli, leek, and green beans in boiling water that is slightly salted. Cook for about 3 minutes, then drain.
- Drain the pasta and return it to the pan with the reserved liquid from the canned salmon. Add the vegetables, parsley and crème fraiche.

- Stir together over medium heat for a minute or so, adding the salmon pieces at the last minute.

Turkey and Lemon Meatballs

Ingredients:

- Turkey (18 ounces, minced)
- Pepper (pinch)
- Salt (pinch)
- Lemon Juice and Zest (1 lemon)
- Olive oil (1 Tablespoon)
- Breadcrumbs (3 Tablespoon, dried)
- Whipped cream (9 fluid ounces)
- Canola Oil (4 Tablespoons)
- Garlic (1 clove, crushed)
- Onion (0.5 small, finely chopped)
- Pine nuts (1 Tablespoon)

Sauce:

- Pasta (11 ounces, ribbons)
- Broccoli (2 heads, cooked, small florets)
- Chicken broth (7 fluid ounces)

Preparation:

- Sauté on medium heat, the garlic, and onions in a small amount of oil for about 10 minutes, until softened.

- Put in a bowl the turkey, cooked onion, pine nuts, zest, olive oil, and a tablespoon of whipped cream and mix together well. Add salt and pepper.
- Roll into 20 balls and then chill.
- Making the sauce requires boiling the broth and lemon juice until reduced to one-third. Add remaining whipped cream and then boil again. The sauce should automatically thicken.
- Add a few more of the broth if the sauce is too thick. Add salt and pepper to taste.
- Toss two or three tablespoons of olive into a skillet. Throw in the meatballs and cook gently for 15 minutes until slightly browned and completely cooked. Drizzle with the lemon sauce.

Sesame-encrusted Salmon

Ingredients:

- Salt (to season)
- Pepper (to season)
- Thai spice (.5 teaspoon)
- Chili sauce (2 tablespoons)
- Asian marinade (2 tablespoons)
- Baby bok choy (150 grams)
- Salmon Fillet
- Sesame seeds (1 tablespoon)

Preparation:

- Coat the non-skin side of the salmon with a mixture of the Thai spice and .5 of the sesame seeds
- Use the olive oil to coat the skillet. Cook the salmon, over medium heat with flesh side down until the sesame seeds are golden or about three minutes.

- Turn the fish over and cook until preferred approximately from one to two minutes.
- Steam the bok choy for 1.5 minutes. Mix the Asian dressing and the chili sauce together, then toss with the vegetables,
- Put the vegetables on a plate, sprinkle with sesame seeds, then top with salmon.

Roasted vegetables with honey and feta cheese

Ingredients:

- Manuka Honey (3 or 4 tablespoons)
- Feta cheese (7 ounces)
- Thyme (4 sprigs)
- Olive oil (6 tablespoons)
- Butternut squash (.5, peeled and cut into cubes)
- Red onions (2, quartered)
- Baby Courgettes (1.2 pounds, diagonally halved)
- Carrots (2 chopped)
- Bell peppers (2 red, sliced thick)

Preparation:

- Preheat the oven to 400 degrees Fahrenheit. Drizzle olive oil on a roasting pan or tin and place the vegetables on it. Season and add the thyme.
- Roast for 40 minutes.
- Cube the feta cheese and add vegetables. Stir thoroughly with honey.
- Return to oven for another five minutes.

Tomato and Mango Curry

Ingredients:

- Rice (cooked, to serve)
- Yogurt (1.25 pints)
- Mango (1 large, firm, skin on and cut into chunks)
- Tomatoes (10.5 ounces, chunked)
- Garlic (3 cloves, chopped)
- Turmeric (2 teaspoons)
- Green chilis (3, halved lengthwise)
- Red onion (1 large, sliced)
- Ginger (2-inch piece, chopped)
- Curry leaves (a handful, fresh or dried)
- Mustard seeds (1 teaspoon, black)
- Sunflower oil (2 tablespoons)

Preparation:

- Heat a large skillet or wok over medium heat. Fry the mustard seeds until they start to pop. Proceed to add the curry, turmeric, garlic, ginger, onion, and chilis.
- Season well.
- Once the onion begins to brown, toss in the mango and tomatoes, and then cook until the tomato softens. Remove from heat immediately and whisk in the yogurt.
- Serve immediately.
- Serve on top of rice.

Creamy Salmon Tagliatelle

Ingredients:

- Pepper (pinch)
- Sour cream and chive dip (.5 of 200g tub)
- Salmon (2 cans, skinless and boneless, flaked)
- Baby spinach (1 bag, washed)
- Tagliatelle (8 ounces)

Preparation:

- Boil salted water in a big saucepan and cook pasta for 10 minutes or until tender. Meanwhile, drain the salmon and pick through any bones or skin. Flake the fish.

- Put the spinach in a colander. When the pasta is done cooking, pour the pasta over the spinach. This will slightly cook the spinach while draining the pasta.
- Return both the spinach and pasta to the pan. Stir in the sour cream dip and flaked salmon. Heat until the salmon is hot.
- Season to taste.

Salmon Stir-Fry

Ingredients:

- Walnut Halves (2 ounces)
- Olive Oil (1 tablespoon)
- Baby spinach (6 ounces)
- Cherry Plum Tomatoes (6, halved)
- Orange juice (1 orange squeezed)
- Avocados (2, peeled, pitted, and sliced)
- Green beans (4 ounces)
- Broccoli (6 ounces)
- Salmon fillets (2, skinned and sliced)
- Soy sauce (2 tablespoons)

- Runny honey (1 tablespoon)

Preparation:

- Combine the orange juice, honey, and soy sauce.
- Heat oil in a wok. Toss in the broccoli then stir-fry for two minutes. After that, the salmon and beans need to be added and stir-fried for an additional two minutes.
- Add the remaining ingredients then continue to cook. Always keep the ingredients moving for another two minutes.
- The vegetables should still be crunchy.
- Add in the orange dressing and heat for another minute. Serve immediately with cooked noodles.

Salmon Bake

Ingredients:

- Parsley (handful, chopped)
- Salt (pinch)
- Pepper (pinch)
- Soya cream (284 milliliters)
- Salmon fillet (600 grams, cut into 1inch thick strips)
- Lemon zest (1 lemon)
- Spinach (150 grams, fresh)
- Broccoli (200 grams, florets)
- Garlic (2 cloves, minced)

- Onion (1 large, sliced)
- Potatoes (907 grams, waxy and unpeeled)
- Margarine (75 grams)

Preparation:

- Preheat oven to 400 degrees Fahrenheit.
- Boil the unpeeled potatoes for nine minutes. Drain the potatoes and then rinse with cold water. Set them aside.
- Melt two-thirds of margarine in a pan, throw in onion, garlic, pepper, and then stir-fry for three minutes. Add in the broccoli. Stir-fry for five minutes.
- Throw in the spinach and cook until the green start to wilt.
- Spray a deep baking dish with cooking oil. Spoon the stir-fry mixture over the base evenly. Put salmon fillets on top of the mixture.
- Drizzle with lemon zest, parsley, and the cream.
- Season to taste.
- Take the skins off the potatoes, then grate the potatoes and top the salmon with the shredded potatoes.
- Bake for 30 minutes.

Egg-fried rice with Mushroom and salmon

Ingredients:

- Lemon juice (.5 lemon)
- Sesame Oil (1 tablespoon)
- Soy sauce (3 tablespoons, low-sodium)
- Eggs (3, beaten)
- Mushrooms (12 ounces, portobello, or shiitake mushrooms)
- Groundnut oil (2 tablespoons)

- Salmon fillets (12 ounces)
- Peas (4 ounces, frozen)
- Jasmin Rice (6 ounces)

Preparation:

- Cook the rice for 10 minutes in salted, boiling water. Add the peas in the last two minutes. Drain in a colander and then set aside.
- In a skillet, add six tablespoons of water with the salmon, bring to boil.
- Cover the fish and simmer for about 8 minutes or until cooked. Transfer to a plate. Take off any skin and flake the flesh.
- Over high heat, heat up a wok and add half of the oil. Whisk the eggs and add them to the wok. Stir until scrambled.
- Transfer to a plate and wipe the wok, then return it again to the heat. Add the rest of the oil.
- Add in the mushrooms then stir-fry until softened for about 2 minutes.
- Toss in the rice, peas, salmon, eggs, soy sauce, and the lemon juice, and then stir to heat. Serve once piping hot.

Coriander and Chickpea Salad

Ingredients:

- Salt (pinch)
- Pepper (pinch)
- Olive oil (60 milliliters)
- Garlic (1 teaspoon, chopped)
- Onion (1 teaspoon)

- Mustard cream (2 teaspoons)
- Lettuce leaves
- Coriander leaves (4 teaspoons, chopped)
- Ceylon Teabags (3 bags)
- Cherry Tomatoes (handful, diced)
- Chickpeas (1 can)

Preparation:

- Put the chickpeas in saucepan filled with water and the teabags. Boil until the chickpeas are cooked and softened.
- Toss the tea bags out, drain and cool the chickpeas.
- Add together the olive oil and mustard cream. Season with salt and pepper. Toss in the tomatoes, onion, garlic, and coriander. Mix well.
- Serve over lettuce.

Beat and Bean Salad

Ingredients:

- Pepper (.25 teaspoon)
- Olive oil (2 tablespoons)
- Salt (.25 teaspoon)
- Garlic (1 teaspoon, minced)

- Thyme (2 teaspoons, chopped)
- White wine vinegar (1.5 tablespoons)
- Parsley (3 tablespoons, chopped)
- Red beets (12 ounces, peeled and wedged)
- Green beans (1 8-ounce package)

Preparation:

- Wrap the beet wedges in microwave-safe parchment paper. Microwave on high for 11 minutes.
- Microwave green beans according to package directions.
- Toss together and whisk the oil, parsley, vinegar, thyme, garlic, salt, and pepper. Add in beans and beets.

Roasted Cauliflower and Oranges

Ingredients:

- Orange (1 whole)

- Sherry vinegar (2 tablespoons)
- Red onion (1 cup, sliced)
- Red pepper (.25 teaspoon, crushed)
- Olive oil (3 tablespoons)
- Cauliflower (4 cups, small florets)
- Salt (.5 teaspoon)
- Orange zest (2 teaspoons)
- Oregano (1 tablespoon)

Preparation:

- Preheat broiler. Add in the olive oil, vinegar, oregano, orange zest, salt, and red pepper. Throw in cauliflower and onion. Toss together.
- Spread the mixture on a baking sheet and line with aluminum foil.
- Broil for 10 minutes, stirring after 4 minutes. Top with orange pieces.

Roasted lemon and parsnips

Ingredients:

- Lemon (1, sliced into wedges)
- Salt (.25 teaspoon)
- Dill (1 tablespoon, chopped)
- Olive oil (1 tablespoons)
- Parsley (.25 cup, chopped)
- Pepper (.25 teaspoon)
- Lemon juice (1 tablespoon)
- Parsnips (1 pound, peeled and sliced thin)

Preparation:

- Preheat oven to 500 degrees Fahrenheit. While the oven preheats, place a cookie sheet on it. Note: Do not take the pan out while preheating!
- Combine the olive oil, lemon juice, pepper, parsnips, and salt. Layout on the baking sheet.
- Bake for ten minutes and then top with parsley and dill.

Conclusion

The benefits of this book will assist you to become more knowledgeable of the healthiest foods on the planet. Superfoods are easily accessible and affordable, and there are many more than you may have thought previously existed. All the superfoods are extremely healthy and are low in calories.

You will not have a problem eating in a super healthy manner because superfoods are, by definition, extremely nutritious.

These recipes are written out and easy to follow. They are all divided into three chapters: breakfast, lunch, and dinner. Breakfasts are all under 400 calories, lunches and dinners are both under 600 calories and they all take less than an hour to prepare.

Thank for making it through to the end of *The Complete Superfoods*. Let's hope it was informative and able to provide you with all the tools you need to achieve your goals whatever they may be.

The next step is to pick your favorite recipe and to try it out!

** Remember to use your link to claim your 3 FREE Cookbooks on Health, Fitness & Dieting Instantly

https://bit.ly/2Lvj2Pm

CPSIA information can be obtained
at www.ICGtesting.com
Printed in the USA
BVHW041812021220
594600BV00023B/292

9 781801 330039